The Dukan Diet

Uncovering The Secrets To Easy Weight Loss

(A Comprehensive Analysis Of The Well-known French Diet)

Antoine Thompson

TABLE OF CONTENT

Dukan Diet Allowed Items.. 1

Positives And Negatives Of The Dukan Diet 10

The First Two Processes 25

Zesty Lemon Pancakes..33

The Guidelines For The First Two Segments............35

Homemade Sugar And Nonfat Icy Yogurt..................44

Chili Ginger Roast Chicken 47

Acidity And Cancer 49

Spicy Meatballs Made Of Sausage And Ground Turkey 53

Steamed Fish Chinese Style 55

Should I Adhere To The Dukan Det? 57

Two Stages Of Weight Reduction 84

Homemade Noodle Broth...88

Foil-Baked Flounder 91

Stabilization 93

Dukan Diet Allowed Items

Despite its rather strict structure, you've presumably deduced that the Dukan diet permits you to consume freely from what has been said so far. As long as you consume only the permitted foods, you have nothing to worry about. The good news is that there is no restriction on how much you can consume. 72 pure proteins derived from various sources (non-fat dairy, seafood, vegetable proteins, seafood, fish, and meat) and 28 vegetables (allowed beginning with the cruise phase) are included on the list of permitted foods. The Dukan diet recommends daily consumption of bran, which is considered an essential component.

The foods that have been incorporated into the Dukan diet are those that the first males to inhabit our planet consumed. During the research phase,

Dr. Dukan identified these foods as containing all the nutrients our bodies require, with a high protein content and low fat and carbohydrate levels. Let's examine the foods permitted on the Dukan diet.

First, there are pure protein sources, which are recommended as early as the attack phase. Lean meat is one of the most essential sources of unadulterated proteins. There are venison, veal chops, veal scaloppini, steak, low-fat bacon, pork tenderloin and loin roast, roast beef, pork chops, lean kosher beef, bison, filet mignon, and beef tenderloin among the recommended foods in this category. When it comes to beef, it is important to remember that ribs should be avoided due to their high lipid content. As for the veal pieces, you must remove all of the flesh before eating them. Low-fat ham and smoked turkey are also permitted, making them the ideal ingredients for a delectable sandwich. You may also consume thin slices of desiccated beef, but avoid cured or smoked hams due to their high fat content.

Regarding poultry, the following foods are recommended: wild duck, turkey, quail, ostrich (steak), low-fat deli (chicken or turkey), fat-free sausage (chicken or turkey), Cornish hen, chicken liver, and chicken. Domestic geese and ducks are prohibited, and for all poultry, the skin must be removed prior to consumption. Due to its high fat content, the outer portion of the wings cannot be ingested. It is also recommended to consume lean game animals, such as pheasant. The lipid content of various chicken segments varies, and you must be aware of this. The chicken breast contains the least quantity of fat, followed by the quadriceps and the wings. Additionally, for the chicken to have a low lipid content, it must be as immature as feasible.

Fish is an excellent source of unadulterated protein, with the following options allowed: Tuna (fresh or canned in water), trout, swordfish, surimi, shark, sea bass, sardines (fresh or canned in water), salmon (smoked salmon is also permitted), red snapper, mahi mahi, mackerel, herring, halibut (smoked), cod, catfish, and arctic char. You might question the selection of cured salmon, particularly given its oily appearance. However, you must remember that the smoked salmon contains significantly less fat than a fat-free fillet, despite its oily appearance. The same holds true for other types of smoked fish, such as halibut, tuna, eel, trout, and haddock. Regarding the fish in a can, this is permissible as long as it was canned in water or tomato sauce.

As for surimi, you're likely aware that it contains slender white fish meat and imitates crab skewers. Numerous controversies surround this product, which is flavored with crab marinade and (not very much) sugar. Even though this product is processed and may contain carbohydrates, its low fat content allows it to be included in a healthy diet.

You may not use oil or butter when preparing fish, but you may use lemon juice, soy sauce, and an abundance of fresh seasonings. As you will see, there are numerous ways to prepare fish, including steaming, roasting, and poaching. Additionally, spices are permitted.

Regarding seafood, the following options are available: squid, shrimp, scallops, oysters, octopus, mussels, lobster, crawfish, crab, and clams. Not only is seafood recommended as a method to add variety to your diet menu, but it is also quite substantial and satisfying.

Tofu, tempeh, soy, soy-based products, vegetarian patties, and seitan are examples of plant-based protein sources. I highly recommend the tofu and seitan due to their exceptionally balanced protein, carbohydrate, and lipid content. The other options are more advisable for vegetarian dieters who do not eat meat or fish. The most prevalent forms of tofu are silken tofu (consistency similar to yoghurt) and firm tofu (consistency similar to semi-soft cheese). On supermarket shelves, you can find various types of tofu, including the herb-flavored, charred, and curry-flavored varieties. Tofu can be used to make dumplings, sausages, and even ravioli, so you have a wide range of options.

You may also ingest dairy products that are fat-free or low-fat, such as sour cream, ricotta, basic Greek yogurt, cream cheese, and cottage cheese. There are no restrictions on the quantity of natural and flavored yogurt. Conversely, the consumption of fat-free fruit yogurt should be restricted. During the assault phase, it is optimal that you avoid them entirely. During the assault phase, you may consume sugar gelatin as well.

Also recommended are whole eggs, including those from chicken, quail, or duck. You may blanch, poach, or make an omelet with the eggs as long as no butter or oil is used. Ensure that the eggs are thoroughly cooked, particularly if you are uncertain about their origin (salmonella risk). Egg substitutes with a reduced lipid content are also permitted. The egg substitutes are available in fresh, refrigerated, and powdered forms. As you will learn in the chapter on recipes, you can combine eggs with seafood (crab in particular), vegetables, or prosciutto. If you have a high cholesterol level, you should limit yourself to three or four egg yolks per week. On the other hand, egg whites, which are the purest natural source of protein, can be consumed without restriction. During the assault phase, you may consume up to two eggs per day. Do not hesitate to attempt the egg white omelet for brunch, as it is a delectable choice.

Beginning with the cruise phase, you are permitted to consume certain vegetables (non-starchy and low in fat). Zucchini, watercress, turnip, tomatoes, spinach, squash, rhubarb, radishes, pumpkin, peppers, shallots, leeks, onions, mushrooms, radicchio, lettuce, kale, green beans, fennel, endive, eggplant, cucumber, celery, cauliflower, carrot, cabbage, Brussels sprouts, beet, bean sprouts, asparagus, and artichoke are among the permitted vegetables.

On the Dukan diet, you are permitted to consume additional ingredients. Certain of them, such as shirataki, may be ingested beginning with the attack phase. Shirataki is an Asian root that can be truly satiating despite its low caloric content; furthermore, its high fiber content means that it can contribute to the enhancement of intestinal motility. There are various forms of Shirataki available, including powder, flour, and emulsion.

Additionally, olive oil is permitted during the cruise phase. However, daily consumption is restricted to one teaspoon. Olive oil is a healthful option because it contains omega-3 fatty acids, polyphenols, and vitamin E, a potent antioxidant. The Dukandiet includes Goji berries beginning with the assault phase. On natural protein days, you are permitted to consume one tablespoon of goji berries, whereas on protein and vegetable days, you are permitted to consume two tablespoons.

The Dukan Diet also encourages hydration, with a variety of beverages recommended for daily consumption. During the assault phase, mineral water with a low sodium content (which has diuretic and cathartic properties) is highly recommended. High-sodium mineral waters should be avoided during the Dukan diet because they can cause water retention and contribute to overall weight gain.

In addition to bottled water, tap water is permitted, and you may consume as much of it as you like, as there are no adverse effects to worry about. You may also consume tea, with the most recommended varieties being green tea (which contains antioxidants) and medicinal tea (particularly during the winter). Diet beverages are recommended because they can help diet adherents get through these periods more easily and reduce their cravings for real sugar.

Positives And Negatives Of The Dukan Diet

Benefits of the diet

Weight reduction

Weight loss is one of the Dukan diet's greatest benefits. The regimen is intended to help obese individuals reduce weight and also emphasizes on preventing weight regain. Thus, the diet reduces the risk of developing obesity-related diseases such as cardiovascular disease, hypertension, elevated blood pressure, type II diabetes, etc.

No muscle loss

Since "protein" is the diet's primary nutrient focus, muscle loss will not be an issue. Protein is primarily responsible for the development and maintenance of robust musculature.

No calorie monitoring

The Dukan diet, unlike other regimens, does not emphasize calorie monitoring. Several diets, such as the zone diet, require the dieter to precisely measure everything they consume. This becomes extremely monotonous and could prompt a person to abandon the task in the middle. That hazard is avoided in the Dukan diet.

No portion control

The diet does not restrict the quantity of food consumed. It is essential to consume only the foods listed on the phase-wise food list, but there is no limit on how much of these foods can be consumed, making it ideal for people who are accustomed to eating large portions.

Simple to follow

The diet is not complicated. It is simple to comprehend and execute. It also provides you with a comprehensive cuisine inventory to choose from and clearly outlines the four phases and their regulations. Folks, it does not get any simpler than that!

Result oriented

Within one or two weeks, you begin to observe a significant weight loss on this regimen. The weight loss is progressive, and you will feel increasingly lighter each month until you reach your ideal weight.

Meats promoted

The diet emphasizes the consumption of lean meats, which is excellent news for meat eaters. As everyone knows, meat is extremely abundant in proteins, and since this is the nutrient that is the primary focus of the diet, it is the most efficient and practical form of ingredient.

celebratory cuisine

The two celebratory meals that are permitted after the consolidation phase are the diet's highlight. The two meals are a welcome change for those who are acclimated to consuming a diet high in unhealthy food. The meals are appropriately referred to as "celebration meals."

Sweeteners

Artificial sweeteners and diet beverages are permitted on the diet. Dukan dieters may consume sweetener-based dishes and diet soda according to their preferences. The additives are suitable for use in confectionery.

Vegetarian-friendly

The diet also encourages the consumption of vegetarian food substances, providing vegetarians with an extensive selection. Although there is not as much variety for vegetarians as there is for non-vegetarians, there is a sufficient selection of vegetables and meat substitutes such as tofu.

Negative aspects of the diet

Deficiencies

Several nutrient deficiencies are caused by the diet, particularly during the assault phase. Since proteins are the primary focus, vitamins A, D, C, and E are not included, which can lead to bone loss. Lack of iron can also cause temporary hair loss and brittle nails, among other symptoms. To combat this issue, Doctor Dukan recommends nutritional supplements.

Not for herbivores

The diet is not suitable for vegans due to the high consumption of meat and the absence of vegan-friendly goods on the food inventories. However, according to the diet's argument, vegans do not inherently need weight loss programs, so it is fair to state that vegans are not included in the diet.

Fatigue

Dietary nutrient restrictions may result in fatigue, which is a feeling of weariness. Carbohydrates are essential for energy maintenance, and a lack of this nutrient can cause mood fluctuations and fatigue in dieters.

Sweeteners and beverages

The diet permits the consumption of artificial sweeteners and cola, which can be viewed as a positive; however, these are not necessarily healthful options and can actually negate the benefits of the diet.

Poor respiration

Bad breath is a significant nutritional concern. Additionally, a high protein intake can cause flatulence and leave a metallic residue in the mouth. The issue with poor odor is at its worst during the assault phase.

Kidney dysfunction

Consistently utilizing body fat as opposed to caloric places an additional burden on the kidneys and liver, which can result in severe harm over time. The extra weight can cause the urine to become darker and emanate a pungent odor.

Withdrawal symptoms

Upon completion of the diet, withdrawal symptoms may manifest. These symptoms may include fatigue, vertigo, and migraines, as the body undergoes many changes and finds it difficult to return to its previous diet.

Expensive

The diet can be a costly endeavor; lean meats can be quite expensive. The diet also requires the consumption of nutritional supplements, which increases the expense. The diet will readily increase your monthly expenditures by several hundred dollars.

elevated triglycerides

The excessive consumption of meat can lead to an increase in cholesterol levels. Despite being lean, all meats contain some fat, which can accumulate over time and clog the arteries. Therefore, the regimen is also unsuitable for those with high cholesterol levels.

Exercise

The diet and exercise are highly interdependent. Many individuals find exercise inconvenient, and the interdependence makes it difficult for them to achieve significant results. Dieters are required to exercise daily from the onset of the assault phase through the conclusion.

gout and chronic constipation

Diets strong in protein significantly increase the risk of developing gout. Gout is a condition in which inflammatory arthritis attacks the extremities. The lack of fiber in the diet can result in severe constipation, necessitating the consumption of at least 9 to 10 glasses of water per day, particularly during the attack phase.

Unhealthy Foods

Due to the exclusion of calorie-dense lipids on the Dukan Diet, weight loss is maximized. You can make your meals nutritious and delectable by experimenting with seasonings, lemon juice, soy sauce, and other marinades to replace the flavor lost by consuming lean meat.

The Dukan Diet excludes processed foods and beverages, thereby eliminating hazardous preservatives. Premade or frozen meals frequently contain added sugar or sodium for flavoring, so omitting them from the diet is beneficial for the heart and will lead to weight loss. Even seemingly healthful processed foods, such as juice, are loaded with added sugar and lack the nourishing fiber of whole, uncooked produce. There is simply no means to determine what ingredients have been added to frozen TV entrees. On the Dukan Diet, you will consume only whole, natural foods for which you can enumerate all of the ingredients.

The absence of carbohydrates is the most evident and extreme aspect of the

Dukan Diet. Grains and carbohydrates are high in calories, simple to metabolize, and devoid of vitamins. Because they are so simple to metabolize, our body processes them rapidly, causing an abrupt rise in blood sugar. This is why carbohydrates are a source of fast energy, but the subsequent energy decline is often detrimental. After a rise in blood sugar, the body responds by rapidly producing insulin to aid in carbohydrate digestion. This results in a depressed mood, mental fogginess, and a lack of satiety, causing us to consume more food in order to feel satisfied again. On the Dukan Diet, the protein- and fiber-rich foods will help you feel satisfied longer, so you won't need to count calories to avoid overeating. Fortunately, the Dukan Diet provides a low-calorie alternative to carbohydrates in the form of Shirataki noodles.

Many individuals are unaware that dairy is loaded with fat and carbohydrates. Adults frequently experience blemishes or digestive issues due to dairy consumption; therefore, reducing or eliminating dairy from the diet can result in healthier skin and more regular digestion. Low- or no-fat dairy that is low in lactose is permitted in moderation on the Dukan Diet.

Fruit is also prohibited during the first two phases of the Dukan Diet. While it is true that fruit contains fiber and vitamins, these nutrients are also present in vegetables and goji berries, which are permitted foods. Many of the vegetables on the list, including kale, spinach, and celery, are high in fiber. Goji berries contain eleven different types of vitamins. Fiber, like protein, is a nutrient-dense substance that will keep you satisfied for longer and reduce your appetite.

In the first two phases of the Dukan Diet, indulgences such as biscuits and chocolate are eliminated because they are high in calories, fat, and lack nutritional value. You will be able to consume them again in the final two phases, but only in limited quantities.

The Dukan diet helps you lose weight in several methods. You eat less because: • You are less hungry due to the appetite-suppressing effect of protein; • You can resist unhealthy foods because you are satiated; • Your body is forced to burn calories differently on a high protein diet because it contains only one of the three nutrient categories.

• Excess water is eliminated from the body rather than being retained and accumulating.

• Because your body must work harder to metabolize and extricate calories from the proteins you consume, you expend more calories.   You consume natural foods as opposed to processed foods containing additives and other undesirable compounds.

The First Two Processes

The Attack Methodology

In a maximum of seven days, the assault procedure causes the weight-watcher to lose two to three kilograms of weight. During this phase, the weight-watcher's metabolism is prepared for the initial phase of the diet. The dieter is permitted to consume protein from 80 different dietary categories.

Depending on the patient's level of obesity, the schedule would vary. It can be manually adjusted or measured throughout the diet's duration. Simply put, the duration of the assault program can be adjusted accordingly.

The primary objective of the assault is to introduce a nutritious diet. The patient will consume only enough food to satisfy appetite. The greatest amount of weight is lost during this process. The body will gradually adapt to the steady rate of weight loss.

The initial days of this phase are the process's most crucial. The dieter must make concessions to his previous food patterns in order to adopt the new routine of following the process. Among the few disadvantages of this regimen, the initial fatigue is notable. However, the condition improves within three days. The patients' fluctuating energy levels prevent them from engaging in vigorous exercise. This program necessitates three whole meals per day, which is another reason for less exercise. It makes the patient feel satisfied, which is crucial for discouraging patients from eating anything other than protein.

In addition to 112 tablespoons of oat bran per day, the following ingredients are recommended for the assault phase:

1. Trimmed beef, rabbit, or veal, excluding the ribcage

Turkey and chicken without skin, as well as the wing tips

3. lean ham, thinly sliced

4. Liver

5. Fresh seafood

Crabs, prawns, and other forms of crustaceans and shellfish

7. Two eggs per day, preferably without the yolk

2% or less reduced-fat dairy products

Non-fructose sweeteners, spices, mustard, vinegar, herbs, onion as a spice, garlic, lemon juice only as a condiment and not as a juice drink, sugar-free ketchup and sugar-free chewing tobacco.

Occasional negative effects of the assault process do, however, manifest. Constipation is one of them because protein-rich diets lack fiber. The Dukan Diet requires the consumption of oat flour for this reason. However, sufficient hydration and wheat bran meal can rectify the issue.

Protein-rich diets can lead to respiratory difficulties, which can be remedied with water. Additionally, sugar-free chewing gels can be useful.

Protein-rich diets can induce dehydration because they stimulate kidney function. To combat this issue, the daily water intake should be increased to 1.5 liters.

As oat bran is a required dietary component, it is recommended to consume it as porridge, a counterpart to yogurt, or as a component of pastries or loaves.

During the assault process, both the physical and nutritional aspects must be maintained. Exercise ought to be minimal. Twenty minutes of walking is adequate.

It is observed that no improvement is discernible after approximately five days. At this stage in the process, the dieter must transition to the subsequent phase, known as the cruise phase. It is advised that the assault procedure not be prolonged.

Simple online research can help you discover additional meals to complement the recommended Dukan Diet foods.

Cruise Period

After the effective completion of the assault phase, the cruise phase would begin. At this point, approximately two pounds or one kilogram should be lost per week. The dieter would partition each meal plan into two five-day portions: (i) unadulterated protein, and (ii) a mixture of protein and vegetables. It is a challenging dietary regimen, so the dieter must be motivated. Alternating between the cuisines on a daily basis is an alternative option. This time, a similar result is obtained, although it is believed that the previous protracted procedure had advantages. During the five-day course of the regimen, for instance, the process of skin tightening is permitted.

The elderly will observe two distinct diets: (i) a two-day protein diet and (ii) a five-day protein diet with vegetables. However, this process is slower than the previous two.

Here is a list of vegetables that should be consumed during the second phase of the aforementioned three regimens.

1. Aubergine

2. Asparagus

3. Artichoke

4. Broccoli 5. Cauliflower

6. Brussels 7. Sprouts

8. Chicory 9. Courgette 10. Celery 11. Leeks

Twelve. cucumber thirteen. French beans

14. Onions 15. Mushrooms

16. Peppers 17. Pumpkins

18. Salad greens 19. Spinach 20. Radicchio 21. Soybeans

22. Radish 23. Tomato 24. Sorrel 25. Swede 26. Swiss chard

These vegetables have substitutes if they are unavailable. Carrots and beetroots can be consumed in tiny amounts alongside the aforementioned vegetables.

At this point in the diet, the dieter may consume two tablespoons of oat bran per day.

At this point, a 30-minute walk is ample for physical activity.

At the conclusion of the cruise phase, the dieter should have reached his target weight. The 15th day of the Dukan Diet program will have passed at this point. The anticipated weight loss during this segment of the program is 16 pounds or 7 kilograms, or roughly 5 kilograms during the attack phase and 2 kilograms during the cruise phase.

Zesty Lemon Pancakes

Ingredients:

- 8 tbsp fat-free yogurt
- 4 tbsp sweetener
- Zest of a lemon
- 2 eggs
- 2 egg whites
- 2 tbsp oat bran

Preparation:

- Beat the egg whites and eggs together in a basin.

- Add oat bran, yogurt, sweetener, and lemon zest to this mixture, stirring well.

•In a non-stick pan, heat a few droplets of oil, making sure it reaches every corner.

•Spread some pancake batter onto the griddle. Cook until bubbles form on the pancake over a medium heat.

•Then, flip the crepe and allow it to continue cooking until it turns brown in color.

•Repeat until all of the mixture has been utilized.

The Guidelines For The First Two Segments.

The Attack Step

During the assault phase, the dieter is programmed to lose between two and three kilograms of superfluous weight within two to seven days. At this stage, the dieter's metabolism is primed for the initial assault of the diet. The patient may consume as much as he desires from sixty-eight varieties of protein-rich foods.

However, it must be noted that the duration may vary depending on the person's current level of obesity. This can be sensed and calculated during the weight loss program. In brief, the number of days spent in the assault phase can be modified as needed.

The primary objective of the attack phase is to establish healthy dietary routines. In addition, starvation issues will be addressed at this level. Here is presumably where the greatest degree of weight loss will be attained. As the relevant activity continues, the body adapts to a more consistent rate of weight loss.

In these early days, the difficulty is at its greatest. The dieter must overcome previous poor eating practices and an unhealthy addiction to certain foods, such as sweets and confectionery. Consider this a warning that, as the body adapts to the program, one may become readily fatigued or weary. Typically, this dissipates in three days. In the majority of cases, an increase in vitality is observed. At this time, vigorous exercise is discouraged, whereas three meals per day appear mandatory. Each supper must be of sufficient size to occupy the stomach. There is no reason to starve. In actuality, the patient must prevent appetite in order to avoid subsequent cravings.

In addition to oat bran, which is required at 1.5 tablespoons per day, the following foods are recommended during the assault phase:

Lean beef, rabbit, or veal without ribcage

Turkey and chicken, minus the skin and outermost portion of the wings.

Ham lean and minimal in fat

4. liver from chicken, veal, or beef,

5. fish of any variety, but not canned with sauce or oil;

Crabs, prawns, and various crustaceans and shellfish,

7. No more than two eggs per day, with as little yolk as feasible.

Low-fat dairy products, which contain less than 2% fat, and

Non-fructose sweeteners, spices, mustard, vinegar, herbs, onion as a spice, garlic, lemon juice as a condiment and not as a juice drink, sugar-free natural ketchup, and sugar-free chewing gum.

Certain consequences during the assault phase may not be desired by proponents. Irritability is one. This is because protein-rich diets typically contain less fiber. Because of this, oat bran is a mandatory component of the Dukan diet from the very beginning. Additionally, consuming adequate quantities of water and incorporating wheat bran into meals will prevent constipation.

Protein-based diets can also result in poor odor, which can be remedied by drinking water. Additionally, sugar-free chewing tissues are desirable.

It should be noted that protein-rich diets can overwork the kidneys and cause dehydration. Therefore, 1.5 liters of water should be consumed daily to counteract this disadvantage.

As previously stated and emphasized, oat bran plays an important role in the overall diet plan. It can be consumed as desired, i.e., in the form of porridge, as a complement to yogurt, or as a component in pastries and other types of bread.

After completing the segment on food consumption, the physical aspect is the next area to be attacked. There is no need for extensive exercise. In fact, it is not recommended at all. A daily walk of twenty minutes will be beneficial.

Assume that after, say, five days, there has been no improvement. In this case, the dieter must proceed to the next phase, the maintenance phase. It is not advised to extend the assault phase.

Regarding the food options permitted by the Dukan Diet, a basic Internet search will yield a wealth of information.

Cruise Period

Following the conclusion of the assault phase, the next step is the cruise phase. The average healthy weight loss per week is approximately two pounds, or one kilogram. In this case, the dieter must alternate between two sets of dietary components on five-day intervals, namely (a) five days of pure protein intake and (b) five days during which the patient consumes a mixture of protein and vegetables. Due to the duration of each interval, the alternative scheme may be too difficult for a dieter who requires a high level of motivation to execute. Therefore, a one-day cadence may be considered as an alternative method for alternating the two food categories. Although some theories assert that a prolonged period for each interval has some advantages, the effects are comparable. Under the five-day intervals, for instance, the epidermis is allowed for shrinkage. Consequently, flabs do not develop.

The recommended pattern for older individuals is (a) two days of unadulterated protein and (b) five days of combined protein and vegetables. Under this procedure, lipids are eliminated at a slower rate than in the two other sets of intervals described in the preceding paragraph.

All three rhythms permit the following vegetables: aubergine, asparagus, artichoke, broccoli, cauliflower, Brussel sprouts, chicory, courgette, celery, leeks, cucumber, French beans, onions, mushrooms, peppers, pumpkins, salad leaves, spinach, radish, soya beans, turnips, tomatoes, spinach, sorrel, swede, and Swiss chard. Naturally, these vegetables have localized equivalents depending on location. Also permitted, but in moderation, are carrots and beets.

Increasing quantities of oat grain continue to be incorporated. Now, the dieter can consume two tablespoons per day.

For the physical component, the patient must walk at a moderate pace for thirty minutes per day.

At the conclusion of the maintenance phase, the dieter should have reached his or her objective or desired weight. At this point, the Ducan Diet program must be fifteen days into its implementation. Under the assumptions considered here, the total weight loss should be approximately seven kilograms or sixteen pounds. Five kilograms of weight loss could have been accomplished during the attack phase, and the remaining two kilograms could have been lost during the cruise phase.

Homemade Sugar And Nonfat Icy Yogurt

Ingredients:

3 teaspoons of sugar-free jelly

3 tablespoons of boiling water

500 grams fat-free natural yoghurt

Instructions:

First, combine the heated water and sugar-free gelatin powder in a small basin until the jelly is completely dissolved and there are no particles at the bottom of the container. Allow two minutes for the mélange to settle. Blend together the yogurt and gelatin syrup in a food processor.

You can also do this with a utensil, but be sure to thoroughly combine the ingredients. This is the basic formula for frozen yogurt. Without an ice cream maker, preparation time is ten minutes and cooking time is four hours. Cooking time with an ice cream maker is less than one hour.

Using an ice cream maker: Pour the mixture of yogurt and gelatin into your ice cream machine and follow the manufacturer's instructions. The cooking time is under an hour.

Without an ice cream maker, place the mixture in the freezer, cover it, and let it set for thirty minutes. Then, remove the container from the freezer and thoroughly combine the contents. Before placing the yoghurt back in the freezer, ensure that all the ice has melted and that the consistency is uniform. Repeat this process every half-hour until the desired consistency is reached, then consume immediately.

Chili Ginger Roast Chicken

INGREDIENTS

3 cloves chopped garlic

1 tsp. paprika

2 tsp. oregano

1 medium whole chicken

1 lemon

1 red chili pepper

1 Tbsp. fresh ginger

INSTRUCTIONS

Start by preheating your oven to 200 degrees Fahrenheit.

Next, divide your lemon in half. Squeeze the fresh lemon juice into the chicken's cavity, then cut the lemon into segments and place them inside as well.

The chicken should be placed in a roasting pan. Using a pointed knife, make several 1 inch-deep slits in the chicken breast.

Now divide your red chile pepper lengthwise and remove the seeds. Cut it into coarse pieces. Place the pepper pieces, ginger, and minced garlic cloves into the incisions in the chicken breast in a random pattern.

Sprinkle paprika and oregano on the exterior of the chicken and press into the skin. Then position in oven.

Depending on its size, chicken must bake for 1 12-2 hours. Ensure liquids are clear prior to removing food from the oven. Sculpt and serve.

Acidity And Cancer

People believe that cancer thrives in acidic environments and that an alkaline diet can treat or even cure cancer.

Despite extensive research, there is no evident relation between food-induced acidosis (increased blood acidity due to diet) and cancer.

Initially, sustenance has little effect on the pH of the blood.

Even though consuming significantly alters the pH of your blood and other organs, cancer cells do not only flourish in acidic environments.

Normal body tissue, which has a pH of 7.4 and is slightly alkaline, is optimal for the growth of malignancy. Multiple studies have demonstrated that cancer cells may flourish in an alkaline environment.

However, the acidity is generated by the lesions themselves, not the surrounding environment. Cancer cells generate the acidic milieu, not cancer cells themselves.

Nutritional acidity and early humans' diet
From an evolutionary and scientific standpoint, the acid-base theory has numerous flaws.

87% of pre-agricultural humans consumed an alkaline diet, according to a study that served as the foundation for the modern alkaline diet.

Half of the pre-agricultural individuals had net alkaline-forming diets, while the other half had net acid-forming diets, according to new research.

Consider how diversified their diet was, given that they lived in diverse climates and had access to a greater variety of nutrients than we do. As humans moved north of the equator and away from the tropics, diets high in acid-forming foods became more prevalent.

About half of hunter-gatherers consumed a diet that was net acid-forming, although modern maladies were likely far less prevalent.

The Alkaline Diet Food List: What to Consume and Avoid

In planning the diet, the pH of individual foods is considered. Despite their somewhat corrosive pH, grains can be consumed for their health benefits due to their diversity. To maintain an alkaline diet, you must avoid acidic foods, limit or eliminate neutrals, and prioritize alkaline foods from the list below.

Spicy Meatballs Made Of Sausage And Ground Turkey

Ingredients:

3 eggs

¼ onion, minced

¼ teaspoon ground black pepper

1 (20 ounce) package bulk spicy Italian turkey sausage

1 (20 ounce) package spicy Italian ground turkey

Directions:

Before making the meatball mixture, preheat the oven to 350 degrees Fahrenheit (175 degrees Celsius).

Add all ingredients to a combining basin and distribute the onion, pepper, and egg evenly throughout the minced turkey and sausage. You may also try incorporating the sausage and minced turkey first, followed by the remaining ingredients. Make rolls of approximately 1.5-inch discs.

Balls are lined up on a baking tray. Bake for 18 to 20 minutes, or until each ball emits fluid.

Steamed Fish Chinese Style

Ingredients:

- spring onion, chopped up
- cherry tomatoes, sliced in 2
- shitaki mushrooms, sliced

- 1 whole fish (for best results use non-oily fish like bream)
- ginger, julienned

Instruction

Rub the fish with salt and pepper. Cut three incisions on each side of the fish, then stuff it with ginger and onion. Alo stuffed fish stomachs. Add tomato, shitaki, and the remaining red onion on top. Add a pinch of light soy sauce, a pinch of Chinese cooking wine, and a few drops of sesame oil. Place in a steamer or wok over boiling water (using a metal rack) and stir-fry. Depending on the size of the fish, it should take 10 to 20 minutes.

Should I Adhere To The Dukan Det?

The Dukan Diet may help you lose weight quickly, but it is not risk-free. The Dukan Diet is a high-protein, low-carbohydrate diet that does not appear to result in any additional weight loss compared to a diet that promotes healthful eating habits. In the final phase of the diet, you are instructed to eat whatever you want, which could lead to the return of unhealthy eating habits. The uuallu typically results in weight regain.

A diet as restrictive as the Dukan Diet will ultimately result in weight loss due to a caloric deficit caused by limited food options, boredom, and lack of enjoyment from eating. Weght loss can be made more effective by making changes that can be maintained for a lifetime, which means that all foods can be enjoyed.

The Dukan Diet does not educate its adherents on the healthy eating habits necessary for long-term weight loss and good health. A diet that is well-balanced will increase the likelihood of:

Be someone you can depend on (sustain).

Be entertaining.

Provide you with all of the essential nutrients for long-term health.

A well-balanced, nutritious diet consists of fruits, vegetables, whole grains, fish, and nuts, as well as a small amount of meat, dairy, and unsaturated fat. This is supported by extensive research and evidence, unlike the Dukan Diet, which lacks evidence to support its long-term safety and efficacy.

What alternatives exist for losing weight?

Other versions of det are available, for instance:

Paleolithis Diet (Paleo Diet)

Atkins Diet

5:2 Diet

There are other methods to change your diet and lifestyle in order to lose weight, such as increasing your physical activity.

You may find additional pamphlets on this table, including:

Obesitu and Overweight

Weight Reduction (Weight Loss)

Orlistat (Weight Loss Drug)

Weight Loss Surgeru

How to Perform a Dukan Diet

The Dukan Diet is one of the few diets that focuses on foods that were consumed during prehistoric times (when humans engaged in more foraging and gathering). It permits a variety of protein-based foods and non-starchy vegetables. According to the diet, both of these foods are essential for rapid weight loss and long-term weight maintenance. The Dukan Diet is relatively easy to adhere to. It provides a list of 100 "allowed" foods during and after the diet. You may consume as much or as little of these substances as you desire. In addition, there are a variety of resources that provide various recipes and resources that make it easier to adhere to the diet. Review each route of the diet, the permitted foods, and the various recipes so that you can successfully adhere to this program.

Talk to uour dostor.

Prior to beginning a weight loss program or diet, it is essential to determine if weight loss is safe and appropriate for you. You must also consult with your physician to determine if the Dukan Diet is appropriate for you.

Make an appointment to see your health insurance specialist. Discuss your desire to lose weight with your physician and seek their advice on how much weight you should shed.

Also consult your dostor regarding the Dukan Det. Ask if the pattern of consuming is inappropriate for you.

It may also be beneficial to ask your doctor for an additional test or weight loss advice. This is crucial if you have a cardiovascular condition such as high blood pressure or diabetes.

If you and your doctor determine that a diet is appropriate for you, ask your doctor for a referral to a dietitian.

Set objectives for yourself.

When beginning a new diet, it is essential to set goals for yourself. Goals can provide a path to follow and can also be encouraging and motivating.

Your weight-loss objectives must be attainable for you to be successful in your efforts. If you don't, you're setting yourself up for failure.

Typically, only one to two rounds per week are suggested. According to health professionals, this is safe and sustainable weight loss.

If your goal is to lose 10 pounds, losing the weight in two weeks is unrealistic. You will need to lose it over the course of 4-5 weeks.

You may also wish to sonder multiple objectives. You can set one long-term objective followed by shorter-term objectives. This can keep you motivated and encouraged during your weight loss journey.

Make your kitchen and rantru ready.

To ensure that you adhere strictly to the Dukan Diet, it is a good idea to prepare your home. Sresfsallu get the kitchen ready; you'll need to tosk ur on permitted foods and sonder dispose of foods you shouldn't eat.

You are permitted to consume 100 "approved foods" on the Dukan Diet. The diet imposes no restrictions on the quantity of these substances. Theu consist of all rroten ourse (such as eggs, lean beef, pork, seafood, ou and tofu rrodust, and low-fat daru). In addition, all vegetables that are not tarshu are permitted.

Print the list of these foods so you can use them to create a grocery list. You can also use the list to ensure that you do not have any prohibited foods in your home.

Consider donating prohibited foods to a food bank or friends, or discarding them if they've already been opened.

Then, take your approved foods list to the supermarket. Stosks that are permitted on the tem uou enjou and the Dukan Det.

Write ur a meal rlan and recipe salendar.

The Dukan Diet does not impose too many restrictions or laws regarding food and meals. However, creating a menu plan can help you determine what you will eat over the course of a week.

Spend some time with your meal rlan. You must possess the approved food list for the astvtu. Plan out what you will consume for breakfast, lunch, dinner, and dessert for one week on the Dukan Diet.

The meal plan can help you save time, plan meals in advance, and reduce extra visits to the grocery store during the week.

Consider purchasing additional resources.

The official Dukan Diet website does not provide many additional resources for dieters. Consider obtaining the following additional resources if you are unsure of how to follow the diet precisely, if you need additional meal ideas, or if you need motivation:

Weight reduction stumbling. The Dukan Diet includes counseling. This is a paid service that may help keep you motivated and on track while you're attempting to lose weight.

Cookbooks. This regimen also includes several publications that you may wish to read. You explain the diet in detail, provide nutritional information, and even provide recipes and meal suggestions.

Blog and email servise. The Dukan Diet website also allows visitors to sign up for weekly emails and follow a daily blog. These blog posts may provide a unique resource, a reading suggestion, or additional motivation.

Methods for Following the Dukan Diet

Adhere to approved recipes and cooking methods.

With a particular diet, it is essential to adhere to prescribed eating and culinary practices. Following arrrorratelu will result in the greatest weight loss.

The Dukan Diet consists of four distinct phases: the Attack, Crunch, Consolidation, and Stabilization phases. Each phase has distinct "allowed foods" and eating routines. Make sure you are aware of the phase you are in so you can adhere to the diet correctly.

The Dukan Diet cookbook recommends low-fat culinary techniques. Use minimal to no additional fat when cooking.

Download or print different recipes that are appropriate for the Dukan Diet. Also, compile a list of recipes you regularly prepare that adhere to the Dukan Diet protocol.

Consume the proper proportion of protein-rich foods.

The Dukan Diet lists 68 servings of lean protein as "allowed foods." You may consume this food in any phase of the regimen. Ensure that you consume only the following types of protein:

Seafood: arstis shar, catfish, cod, flounder, grourer, haddosk, halibut and smoked halibut, herring, mackerel, mahi mahi, monkfish, orange roughy, perch, red snapper, salmon or smoked salmon, sardines (fresh or canned in water), sea bass, shark, sole, surimi, swordfish, tilaria, trout, tuna (fresh or sanned in water), clams srab, crawfish, sraufish, lobster, mussels, ostorus, ousters, ssallors, shrimr and squid.

Poultru: egg, chicken, chicken liver, Cornish hen, fat-free turkey and chicken sausages, low-fat chicken or turkey deli segments, otrsh teak, ual, turkey, and wild dusk.

Red meats and rork: beef tenderloin, filet mignon, buffalo, extra-lean ham, extra-lean Kosher beef hot dogs, lean senter-sut rork shors, lean slises of roast beef, rork tenderloin, rork loin roast, redused-fat bason (i.e. senter sut belly bason, whish is leaner than regular bason), steak (flank, sirloin, London broil), veal shors, veal ssallorini and venison.

Vegetarian rrotein: seitan, sou foods and veggie patties, temreh and tofu.

Dairy products include fat-free cottage cheese, fat-free sour cream cheese, fat-free milk, fat-free Greek yogurt, fat-free risotto, and fat-free our cream.

The subsequent phase is called voyage.

Dr. Dukan calls the subsequent phase "The Cruise phase," and during this phase, dieters continue to consume high-protein dishes while increasing their vegetable consumption to 28 servings per day.

The strategy calls for alternating days of protein-only consumption with days of protein and vegetables consumption. And you continue to participate in the Cruise program until you have achieved your desired weight loss.

Here are just a few of the 28 recommended vegetables:

Additionally, asparagus, artichokes, and fennel are included.

French beans, aubergine, scallions, and beetroot

broccoli, cabbage, cauliflower, and mushrooms are vegetables.

The four vegetables include pumpkin, bell peppers, carrots, and celery.

This dish consists of tomato, lettuce, and swede.

Examples of a day's worth of protein and vegetables during the Attack phase are...

The morning meal consists of low-fat yogurt. The Dukan crepe

Identical to the prior procedure.

To make a rapid gazpacho for lunch, blanch four tomatoes for thirty seconds in scalding water before skinning, deseeding, and cubing them. 1 red pepper and 1 green pepper should be grilled for 10 to 15 minutes, until charred. After allowing the peppers to cool in a plastic bag, the skin and seeds should be removed, and the peppers should be divided into segments. Place the tomatoes and peppers in a blender along with two peeled, seeded, and diced cucumbers and some mint. Blend until creamy. Serve cooled after adjusting the seasoning to your preference.

Dinner will comprise of chicken with mushrooms and will require 600g of very thinly sliced button mushrooms. Place them in a non-stick casserole dish and drizzle several tablespoons of lemon juice over the top. Add salt and pepper, cover the vessel, and cook over low heat until all of the liquid has evaporated. It is necessary to drain and store the water. Begin by browning one diced onion in a casserole dish with a small amount of water. 800 grams of diced chicken breasts; two minced tomatoes; mushrooms; two chopped garlic cloves; 250 milliliters of low-sodium chicken stock; salt and pepper Prepare over low heat while covered for twenty minutes.

The third phase is called consolidation.

In addition to the original list of 100 natural foods, the Dukan diet permits a greater diversity of foods once you have reached your ideal weight.

According to Dr. Dukan, "the third stage is the Consolidation phase, during which you may reintroduce fruit, bread, cheese, and starchy foods, in addition to two celebration meals per week."

This means that on one night per week, you are free to consume whatever you want, regardless of the consequences (within reason). Throughout the final phases of the consolidation period, this increases to two evenings per week. As part of your efforts to achieve your weight loss objectives, you will continue to consume only protein on Thursdays for the foreseeable future.

Multiplying the number of pounds lost by five will provide an estimate of how long the Consolidation diet will be necessary. For instance, 7lb x 5 Equals 35 days.

The following are guidelines for consuming during the consolidation period:

Consume an optimal quantity of protein and vegetables daily, with the exception of Thursdays, when you should consume only protein.

1 portion of fruit per day, excluding high-sugar fruits such as bananas, grapes, cherries, and preserved fruits. The three finest fruits are considered to be apples, watermelons, and papayas.

You should consume two slices of whole-grain bread with reduced-fat butter every day.

One portion (40 grams) of firm cheese daily; no blue cheese, goat cheese, or other soft or molten cheeses.

During the first half of the Consolidation phase, consume one serving per week of carbohydrate foods such as pasta or rice, and then increase that to two servings per week during the second half. Consider linguine and pasta with tomato sauce. There are numerous other options, including chickpeas, lentils, couscous, polenta, and potatoes.

During the first half of your Consolidation period, you should allow yourself some leeway and reward yourself with a night out or a "special" meal. During the second half of the term, you should increase this number to two. You are free to savor whatever you wish with your dinner tonight.

The fourth stage is referred to as stabilization.

The overwhelming majority of labor-intensive work has been completed. You may now ingest food and beverages on a regular basis while adhering to a few of Dr. Dukan's recommendations.

"Finally, there's the Stabilization phase," he says, clarifying that during this time, you can consume whatever you want without fretting about accumulating weight, so long as you adhere to three fundamental rules.

Utilizing the essential foods from the era of consolidation, "adopt a safety platform"

"Thirty milliliters of oat bran once per day for the rest of your life."

"Make it a rule that every Thursday is a protein-only day."

Even though this is the last period, it is still advised to exercise. The method suggests taking the stairs instead of the elevator and exercising twenty minutes per day.

Additionally, it is essential to consume the recommended daily amount of water, which is 1.5 liters.

What is the maximum amount of weight an individual can anticipate to lose on the Dukan diet?

Certain studies indicate that those who adhere to the Dukan diet may lose as much as two and a half stones of weight.

A cohort of women on the regimen was observed for eight to ten weeks in a study conducted in Poland. In addition, they determined that the average weight loss documented was "approximately 15 kg."

According to Dr. Dukan, "many people have lost a significant amount of weight on the plan and by eating the Dukan diet meals." "How much weight you need to lose and how much weight you want to lose are directly proportional to one another."

According to the Dukan diet, your true weight is "the weight you can achieve without suffering, without compromising your happiness or your health," as well as the weight you can maintain for an extended period of time without excessive exertion, starvation, or dieting.

This ideal weight takes into account the individual's gender, age, and height, among other factors. Plus your heaviest and weakest weights throughout your lifetime.

Two Stages Of Weight Reduction

The Dukan diet gets you off to a decent start by allowing you to consume as much of the permitted foods as you want while losing a respectable amount of weight. The cruise segment then provides additional dining options. Both phases necessitate getting out of a chair and beginning a straightforward exercise program, such as walking.

Attack

Some refer to this phase as Pure Protein (PP). In addition to drinking plenty of water and taking oat bran every day, you may consume as much of 68 different types of lean protein as you please. These include chicken, extra-lean ham, lean roast beef or pork tenderloin, turkey, catfish (not fried), cod, flounder, shrimp, tofu, fat-free cottage cheese and yogurt, veggie burgers, eggs, and sugar-free gelatin. Shirataki noodles, which are made from vegetables, are permitted as well. As with other ketogenic diets, this high-protein, low-carb approach compels the body to obtain its energy from fat rather than carbohydrates.

At the beginning of a diet, it is exciting to see the pounds fall off. However, individuals frequently report feeling fatigued and disoriented at this stage. The ketones your body produces while consuming fat will leave you with a parched mouth and foul breath. Constipation is the only other common negative effect reported during the Attack phase, and oat bran is intended to prevent it. Daily consumption of at least 6 containers of water helps eliminate toxins from the body and, in conjunction with oat bran, maintains digestive health.

How long is the Attack phase active? Typically between 2 and 5 days, according to the Dukan diet's website. Those who have more weight to lose can anticipate to devote one week to the process. In preparation for the next phase of the Dukan diet, you should also begin walking or another simple exercise program during this period.

Cruise

Here is where you lose the most weight. Carrots, green beans, lettuce, mushrooms, okra, tomatoes, and squash are currently acceptable. You are permitted to consume as much of 100 foods, both protein and vegetables, as you can tolerate without gaining weight. This varies depending on the individual. For instance, a person may begin to acquire weight after consuming salmon.

That eliminates salmon from the menu, but there are plenty of other seafood options.

Regardless of the allowed foods, you must alternate pure protein days with protein and vegetable (PV) days. This can be as straightforward as 1 PP/1 PV or as complex as 5 PP/5 PV if you need to lose a significant amount of weight. You will continue to consume daily oat bran and drink copious amounts of water, in addition to exercising.

The excellent news is that you can now consume up to 1 teaspoon of olive oil per day. This increases your culinary options. Those who have subscribed to paid coaching have access to hundreds of recipes, but it is often possible to modify a favored recipe so that it works with your current diet stage. Two Dukan recipes, one for the Attack phase and the other for the Cruise phase, are provided below.

Homemade Noodle Broth

Ingredients:

1 package of shirataki noodles

Salt and spices to taste

½ pound of extra-lean beef, not ground

Preparation:

Cut the beef into ¼-inch cubes. Drain the shirataki noodles and rinse them under cold water for 10-15 seconds. Dry them on a paper towel.

Instructions:

Place approximately 212 cups of water and beef in a saucepan and bring to a simmer. Reduce heat and simmer beef for approximately 20 minutes, or until cooked through. To shirataki noodles, add seasonings. Once more bring to a boil, then immediately reduce heat and simmer for two to three minutes. Serve.

Foil-Baked Flounder

Ingredients:

1 tomato, sliced

1 tsp olive oil

Salt and pepper

One 6-ounce fillet of flounder

1 small onion, diced

Instructions:

Heat oven to 325 degrees Fahrenheit. In a nonstick skillet, heat the olive oil and sauté the onion until translucent. On a paper towel, drain.

Place flounder on a sheet of aluminum foil measuring 12 by 6 inches. Cover with onion and tomato, then season with pepper and salt. Additionally, lemon juice or other seasonings may be used. Wrap the food in aluminum foil and secure the edges.

Bake the envelope for 20 to 25 minutes. Remove from oven, allow to rest for 5 minutes, then serve.

Stabilization

This phase of the regimen was devised for Pierre Dukan's first book, "I Don't Know How to Lose Weight," which was a best-seller in France. There are no longer any dietary restrictions; however, you should adhere to the Nutritional Staircase and use common sense.

Inventive but pragmatic

The Dukan diet website states, "Theoretically, there are no more forbidden foods during the Stabilization phase; you can eat whatever you want, but in practice, your new way of eating must be regulated to prevent weight regain."

Self-control is what is meant when the term "control" is used, despite the fact that many people react negatively when they hear the word. You can accomplish

93

that. You've had a great deal of practice and your new dietary patterns are well-established at this point. You have discovered how much better you feel and appear when you adhere to the general principles of this high-protein, low-fat, and low-carbohydrate diet. You are able to indulge in an occasional Celebration Meal without entirely "falling off the wagon." Just maintain a healthy diet and exercise regimen. Whenever possible, take advantage of other opportunities to remain in shape, such as taking the stairs instead of the elevator.

In addition to exercise, you will continue to consume daily oat bran and reserve one day per week for pure protein. This should occur on the same day each week because it is more convenient. If you find yourself gaining weight once more, increase the number of days in the Attack phase.

Maintaining weight loss for life

The focus of your diet will now be on protein, with only minor quantities of fat and carbohydrates included. You are no longer required to select extra-lean cuts of meat, but it's still a good idea to remove excess fat and discard poultry skin. Continue to use nonstick implements and culinary powders to reduce cooking lipids. Choose more vegetables from the lower tiers of the Nutritional Staircase, but a few starchy ones are acceptable as well. In addition to potatoes and maize, you now have access to an extensive selection of carbohydrates. Among these are fruits, grains, and bread.

Long-term adherence to diet and exercise is significantly facilitated by social support. There are many people who want to hear your success tales and who can also relate to the obstacles and struggles you have faced (and may continue to face). Investigate local and online Dukan diet support groups. Those who have previously used weight-loss counseling to reach the Stabilization phase may also purchase coaching through the Dukan diet website. These coaches will provide you with weekly instructions in addition to suggestions, encouragement, and other tools to stay on track.

7- Future for a Dukanar

Now let's get to the crux of the matter.What the Dukan diet holds for a person after undergoing all these weeks of training.It is possible to tell a lengthy, detailed narrative, but I would like to highlight certain points.

The adherent of the Dukan diet can eliminate the obesity and stomach issues that have plagued him/her for a very long time. Therefore, there is no hearing of street noises and no tummy-pointing from those slender and intelligent females.

The Dukan diet is not merely a matter of altering one's diet and engaging in a few exercises; rather, it is a significant means of altering one's lifestyle. You can now continue the tradition of regular exercise and remain physically fit for the remainder of your life if you do so.

⬜If you are overweight and shy away from people out of fear of being dubbed "Fat Notty," the time has come for you to stand in front of that multitude and ask them directly, "Who is one?"You have lost weight and gained strength and are now ready to confront the world with renewed self-assurance.

If you are a student, teacher, or computer scientist who is becoming increasingly sluggish with time, the Dukan diet can do the work for you. You can move with complete assurance and dexterity.For anyone observing you, a role model is someone who is industrious, devoted, and courageous.

The Dukan diet is a method of learning through practical application. It is similar to a new text with so many practical examples. And if you work on these practicals over time, you will improve.

The process teaches you self-resistance, perseverance, and the sheer will to advance. It instructs you on how to overcome your interior desires and proceed. It teaches you how to survive when you have no unique supplies. It teaches Hard labor as the key to Success!

8- Why You Will Never Forget Dukan Diet

Now that we have provided a comprehensive description of the Dukan Diet, including its contents, recipes, and exercises, we are in a position to answer the question, "Why will you never forget the Dukan diet?"

The answer is straightforward. As the proverb goes, "Never forget the person who did something for you in life, and never forgive the person who did nothing for you in life."Since the Dukan diet helps a person achieve his goals, it is necessary to not only adhere to it during the diet plan, but also to continue working on it throughout your life.

It is focused on results. It's life-altering. It is a significant step toward experiential learning. It is a powerful method for a person to determine his genuine capabilities. Rather than consuming fatty foods and sitting in a chair all day, this is the most natural way to exist. It is the way to gain conviction in oneself. It is a procedure for determining aptitude. It is about establishing objectives and then contending with all your might to achieve success.So I ask you a question .How could you forget?

The paleo diet is based on the eating habits of prehistoric humanity. Numerous studies indicate that obesity is a consequence of the agricultural revolution. Processed foods strip plants of their nutrients and replace them with useless calories. According to proponents of the Paleo diet, the human body has not yet evolved to metabolize modern foods, resulting in a variety of health complications such as obesity.

How it operates

The Paleo diet is more of a lifestyle than a weight loss program. People who choose this diet can also anticipate a reduction in cardiovascular disease risk and an improvement in athletic performance.

Meats

Meats, including seafood, are the primary components of the paleo diet.

However, only flesh from animals raised organically should be used. This means that these animals are only permitted to consume foods that they would normally consume in the outdoors. Additionally, fish should be captured in the outdoors.

Vegetables

In general, paleo dieters are only permitted to consume uncooked vegetables. Not that Paleo insists on raw food consumption, but you should be able to consume it fresh. As with meat, only organically grown vegetables are permitted on the paleo diet.

Fruits

Fruits are permitted on the Paleo diet, but those attempting to lose weight should limit their intake of sweetened fruits.

Seeds and nuts

People who want to lose weight are advised to consume no more than four ounces of nuts and seeds per day. The Paleo diet prohibits both peanuts and legumes.

Water and tea are the only permitted beverages on the Paleo diet. Sugary beverage consumption is strongly discouraged.

Pros:

The Paleo diet is considered one of the cleanest regimens available. Paleo diet is abundant in vitamins and nutrients. Additionally, it eliminates processed foods and is gluten-free. The proponents of this diet also assert that it can increase vitality levels.

Paleo diet is extremely difficult to adhere to. Plants and animals raised organically are difficult to locate and frequently expensive. It also limits an excessive amount of fruits and vegetables. Those who are not accustomed to an organic lifestyle will find the Paleo diet to be extremely difficult.

THE DUKAN DIET MAY BE A HEALTHY OPTION FOR YOU.

The United States Department of Agriculture (USDA) dietary recommendations include calorie recommendations and dietary guidelines for a healthy, balanced diet.11 As a high-protein diet that also restricts carbohydrates and healthful fats, the Dukan Diet does not comply with federal dietary guidelines.

Based on the most recent research, the USDA recommends 5 1/2 ounces (approximately 3 servings) of red meat per day for a 2,000-calorie diet. The Dukan Diet consists of a week of eating only protein, followed by alternating days of eating only carbohydrates.

For utanable weght lo, mny health and nutrition exrert recommend counting calories and sreatng a utanable salore deficit, which means ingesting fewer calories than you are consuming. Use this salsulator to determine uour dailu salorie needs to meet uour goals.

Due to the restrictive nature of the Dukan Diet and its effect on animal reproduction, this diet plan is not recommended for long-term weight control and overall health because it does not adhere to USDA guidelines. In addition, the Dukan Diet emphasizes the significance of healthy carbohydrates and good fats as components of a balanced diet.

THE ESSENTIALS OF A HEALTHY, WELL-BALANCED DIET

Health Benefits Although proponents of the Dukan Diet assert that it is an effective weight-loss plan, many individuals find it too restrictive and difficult to adhere to. It is high in protein and low in carbohydrates and lipids, and research indicates that a high-protein diet can lead to nutrient deficiencies and health problems, including sardiovascular disease.

The Health Rk

The main concern with the Dukan Diet and excessive protein consumption is that the liver and kidneys must work extra hard to process the burrodust of protein metabolm, and there is a limit to how much protein the kidneys can process.3 Dr. Dukan claims that drinking a lot of water will solve the problem, but he does not provide any scientific references to support this claim.

In addition, certain "fact" statements in "The Dukan Diet" are either false or highly debatable. For instance, Dr. Dukan refers to the sarbohudrates in root vegetables and whole grains as "slow sugar," meaning that they are broken down into sugar at a slower rate than refined grains and sugar. However, this is not accurate. The wau a food elevates manu variable blood sugar levels.12 A claim that is not supported by evidence that the combination of water and rure rrotein has a negative effect on sellulite.

How often should you exercise on the Dukan Diet?

It is required. Start walking according to Dukan's horse exercises: 20 minutes per day in Attask, 30 to 60 minutes in Cruise, 25 minutes in Conoldation, and 20 minutes in Permanent Stabilization. Dukan also provides information on toning your chest, shoulders, arms, and butt.

Samrle Short-Sleeved Lt

If you decide to follow the Dukan Diet, you will spend the majority of your time in the Cruising Phase, which is more relaxed than the Attainment Phase but more restrictive than the Consolidation and Stabilization Phases. The following list outlines the essentials you'll need during the Crusade Phase. Note that this is not an exhaustive list, and you may be able to find foods that work better for you.

Cruise Phase

Non-fat dairy products (milk, yogurt, cottage cheese) Lean protein (beef, pork, veal, venison, buffalo, knle roultru, fish, shellfish)

Tofu, tempeh, and etan Liver, kdneu, and tongue as organ meats

Cruciferous vegetable (broccoli, cabbage, broccoli, and Brussels sprouts)

Other vegetables (bell rerrer, eggrlant, radishes, green beans, spaghetti uah, tomatoes, mushrooms, artichokes, asparagus, cucumbers, and celery).

Leafu greens (srinash, kale, lettuses)

Eggs with Onions, Leeks, and Shallots

Oat bran

EXAMPLE DIETARY PLAN

During the Cruise Phase, uou will alternate between "Pure Protein" daus and "Protein/Vegetable" daus. This three-dau meal plan provides suggestions for a few meals on the Cruise Phae. Note that some Pure Proten diets include a portion of a high-protein vegetable for nutritional balance. If you choose to adhere to the eating plan, there may be other dishes that better suit your tastes and preferences.

Dau 1: Pure Protein Breakfast: 2 scrambled eggs, 2 turkey bacon strips, and 1/2 ounce of low-fat cottage cheese

1 serving of tempeh tr stir-fry; 1 serving of cauliflower rice

Dinner: 3 ounses grilled shisken breast; 1 sur roasted The Bruel rrout

Dau 2: Protein/Vegetable

Breakfast: Baked Eggs with Kale and Tomatoes; eight ounces of seltzer.

1 serving of warm sriracha salad With Bacon Vinaigrette

Dinner: four ounces of oven-baked salmon with herbs and one ounce of oven-roasted araragu

Day 3: Pure Protein Breakfast: 1 medium size breakfast sausage; 2 eggs over easu

1 serving of Sticky Baked Tofu with hratak noodles for lunch (omit brown sugar).

4-ounce serving of beef liver and scallions; 1 sur cooked brossol'

MEAL PLAN EXAMPLES FOR THE PHASES

The following are sample meal plans for the first three phases of the Dukan diet. Diet:

Attask Phase Breakfast

Non-fat cottage cheese containing 1.5 tablespoons (9 grams) each of oat bran, cardamom, and sugar.

Coffee or tea with nonfat milk and sugar Substitute water for lunch Sandwich with roast beef

Shratak noodles braised in bouillon.

Diet gelatin

Served tea

Dinner

Slim teak and hrmr

Diet gelatin

Coffee or tea sweetened with nonfat milk and sugar substitute.

Water

Cruise Phase

Breakfast

Three eggs scrambled

Cubed tomatoes

Breakfast Coffee with nonfat milk and sugar substitute Water Lunch Grilled salmon on mixed greens with low-fat vinaigrette

Greek yogurt, 2 tablespoons of oat bran (12 grams), and sugar substitute

Isinglass tea Dinner Baked salmon fillet Steamed broccoli rabe and cauliflower Diet ice cream

Coffee sweetened with nonfat milk and sugar substitute.

Hydrologic Consolidation Phase

Three-egg breakfast omelet with 1.5 ounces (40 grams) of cheese and greens.

Coffee with nonfat milk and sugar replacement

Water Lunch Turkeu Sandwich on two slices of whole-wheat bread with 1/2 ounce (81 grams) of cottage cheese, 2 tablespoons (12 grams) of oat bran, cinnamon, and sugar substitute

Intended tea dinner Roat work

Grilled zucchini 1 medium arrle

Desaf coffee with nonfat milk and sugar substitute water Meals on the Dukan

Diet consist of an abundance of meat, vegetables, oat bran, tea, and coffee.

IS IT SUPPORTED BY EVIDENCE?

There is limited research available on the Dukan Diet. However, one study of Polish women who followed the Dukan Diet revealed that they consumed approximately 1,000 calories and 100 grams of protein per day while losing 15 kilograms in 8–10 weeks.

In addition, numerous studies demonstrate that other high-protein, low-carb diets have substantial weight loss benefits.

Multiple factors contribute to the beneficial effects of running on weight.

One of the calories consumed during gluconeogenesis, the process by which protein and lipids are converted into glucose when carbohydrates are restricted and protein consumption is high.

Your body's metabolic rate increases significantly more after eating protein than after eating carbohydrates or fat, leaving you feeling replete and satisfied.

In addition, protein decreases the hunger hormone ghrelin and increases several satiety hormones, causing you to consume less food.

However, the Dukan Diet differs from other high-carb diets in that it restricts both carbohydrates and lipids. It is a low-carb, low-sugar, and low-fat diet.

The rationale for fat loss on a low-carb, high-protein diet is not supported by scientific evidence.

In one study, subjects who consumed fat alongside a high-protein, low-carbohydrate meal burned an average of

69 more calories than those who avoided fat.

The Dukan Diet's initial stages are also low in fiber, despite the fact that a daily serving of oat bran is required.

1.5–2 tablespoons (9–12 grams) of oat bran contain less than 5 grams of fiber, which is a very small amount that does not contribute to the health benefits of a high-fibre diet.

In addition, several healthful sources of fber, such as avocados and nuts, are not permitted on the Dukan diet because they are too high in fat. Although no ualtu tude have been conducted on the Dukan det telf, anecdotal evidence points to a high-protein, low-carbohydrate approach to weight loss.

Is it secure and viable?

The Dukan Det's afetu has not been studied.

However, there are numerous concerns about high protein intake, particularly its impact on bone and kidney health.

In the past, it was believed that a high protein intake could cause harm to the kidneys.

However, recent research has shown that high-protein diets are not detrimental to healthy kidneys.

Those prone to developing kidney stones will see their condition worsen if they consume an excessive amount of protein.

As long as high-rotaum vegetables and fruits are included in a high-protein diet, bone health will not decline.

Recent research indicates that high-protein diets have a positive effect on bone health.

Before commencing a high-protein diet, those with kidney disease, gout, liver disease, or any other serious illness should consult a physician.

Keep in mind that the diet's intricate rules and restrictive nature may make it difficult to adhere to.

Although most people will lose weight during the first two weeks, the "pure protein" diet is extremely restrictive.

The diet also discourages high-fat foods, which are generally unhealthy. Incorporating animal and plant-based fats makes a low-carb diet healthier, more pleasurable, and easier to maintain over time.

The Dukan Diet is undoubtedly safe for the majority of people, but those with certain medical conditions may wish to avoid it. Its emphasis on high-fat diets may be detrimental to your health.